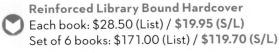

Reinforced Library Bound Hardcover
Each book: $28.50 (List) / **$19.95 (S/L)**
Set of 6 books: $171.00 (List) / **$119.70 (S/L)**

Anywhere Multi-use eBooks
Each eBook: **$35.95**
Set of 6 eBooks: **$215.70**

Battling COVID-19 ©2021   **6 titles**   Print Se

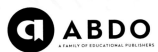

ABDO
A FAMILY OF EDUCATIONAL PUBLISHERS

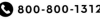 **800-800-1312**   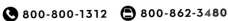 **800-862-3480**   A

T4-AJZ-178

BATTLING COVID-19

Living Apart, TOGETHER

American Life during COVID-19

MARIE BENDER

Checkerboard Library

An Imprint of Abdo Publishing
abdobooks.com

abdobooks.com

Published by Abdo Publishing, a division of ABDO, PO Box 398166, Minneapolis, Minnesota 55439. Copyright © 2021 by Abdo Consulting Group, Inc. International copyrights reserved in all countries. No part of this book may be reproduced in any form without written permission from the publisher. Checkerboard Library™ is a trademark and logo of Abdo Publishing.

Printed in the United States of America, North Mankato, Minnesota
102020
012021

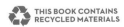

Design: Sarah DeYoung, Mighty Media, Inc.
Production: Mighty Media, Inc.
Editor: Jessica Rusick
Cover Photograph: Shutterstock Images
Interior Photographs: Eden, Janine and Jim/Flickr, p. 7; Glenn Beitz/Flickr, pp. 6 (bottom), 15; Imgorthand/iStockphoto, p. 17; Keith Tsuji/Getty Images, p. 21; Lance Cheung/USDA/Flickr, p. 11; Lorie Shaull/Flickr, pp. 7 (top right), 25; Martin Rickett/AP Images, p. 23; Shutterstock Images, pp. 5, 6, 9, 19, 26, 27, 29
Design Elements: Shutterstock Images

Library of Congress Control Number: 2020940236

Publisher's Cataloging-in-Publication Data
Names: Bender, Marie, author.
Title: Living apart, together: American life during COVID-19 / by Marie Bender.
Other title: American life during COVID-19
Description: Minneapolis, Minnesota : Abdo Publishing, 2021 | Series: Battling COVID-19 | Includes online resources and index
Identifiers: ISBN 9781532194313 (lib. bdg.) | ISBN 9781098213671 (ebook)
Subjects: LCSH: COVID-19 (Disease)--Juvenile literature. | Hand washing--Juvenile literature. | Social distance--Juvenile literature. | Social media--Juvenile literature. | Hygiene--Juvenile literature.
Classification: DDC 302.231--dc23

Contents

The COVID-19 Pandemic

In late 2019, people in Wuhan, China started getting sick with a new disease. Scientists soon discovered the disease was caused by a new coronavirus. The new disease was named COVID-19. Within months, it had spread around the world. On March 11, 2020, the **World Health Organization (WHO)** declared COVID-19 a **pandemic**.

The virus that causes COVID-19 passes easily from one person to another. So, people took action to slow its spread. World leaders told people to stay home when possible. These orders were called stay-at-home orders. Leaders also asked people to practice social distancing. This meant avoiding large gatherings and staying at least six feet (2 m) away from others in public.

Social distancing and stay-at-home orders changed American life. These changes were often challenging. But Americans soon learned how to live apart, together.

WHAT IS A CORONAVIRUS?

Coronaviruses are a large group of viruses that cause **respiratory** illnesses. Most coronaviruses exist only in animals. However, several have spread from animals to humans. The coronavirus discovered in Wuhan is called severe acute respiratory syndrome coronavirus 2 (SARS-CoV-2). It causes a disease called coronavirus disease 2019, or COVID-19. COVID-19 spreads when saliva droplets pass from person to person. This can happen when someone coughs, sneezes, sings, breathes, or talks. Most people with COVID-19 do not suffer serious **symptoms**. But some people develop life-threatening problems. Because of this, the virus is viewed as a threat to world health.

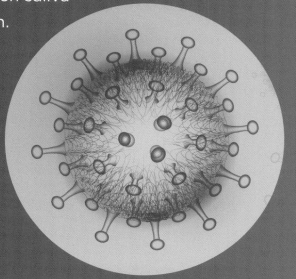

TIMELINE

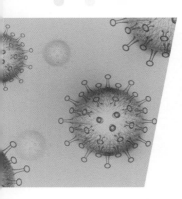

LATE 2019

People in Wuhan, China, get sick with a new disease. It is later named COVID-19.

MARCH 12, 2020

The National Collegiate Athletic Association cancels its athletic championships, including the March Madness tournaments.

MID-MARCH 2020

Most US schools close. Many soon begin holding virtual lessons.

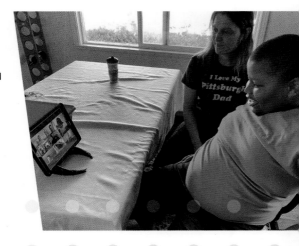

MARCH 11, 2020

The World Health Organization (WHO) declares COVID-19 a pandemic. The National Basketball Association suspends its season.

MAY 2020

Many states begin easing stay-at-home orders, allowing businesses to reopen with safety measures in place.

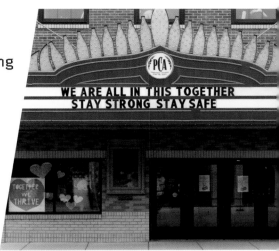

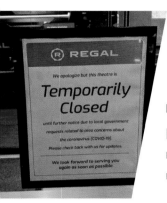

EARLY APRIL 2020

Most US states are under stay-at-home orders.

MARCH 19, 2020

California governor Gavin Newsom issues the first stay-at-home order in the United States.

MAY 18, 2020

More than 1.5 million Americans have been infected with COVID-19. Nearly 90,000 have died.

LATE JUNE 2020

Some states pause reopening as COVID-19 cases increase.

FALL 2020

Some US students go back to school for in-person learning. Other US students continue to attend school from home.

Sheltering at Home

The first stay-at-home order in the United States was in California. Governor Gavin Newsom issued it on March 19, 2020. By early April, most other states were under similar orders. The orders required all **nonessential** businesses to close. These businesses included shopping malls, movie theaters, and gyms.

Millions of people who worked at nonessential businesses lost their jobs. Many other people were able to work from their homes. Schools also closed during the COVID-19 **pandemic**. So, many students attended school online from home as well.

Under stay-at-home orders, officials asked people to only leave their homes for essential travel. This meant people could go to stores for groceries, medicine, and other necessities.

STEM CONNECTION

Face masks are worn over the nose and mouth. They help contain droplets that fly from people's mouths and noses when they cough, sneeze, or talk. These droplets can contain the virus that causes COVID-19. So, wearing face masks helps limit COVID-19's spread.

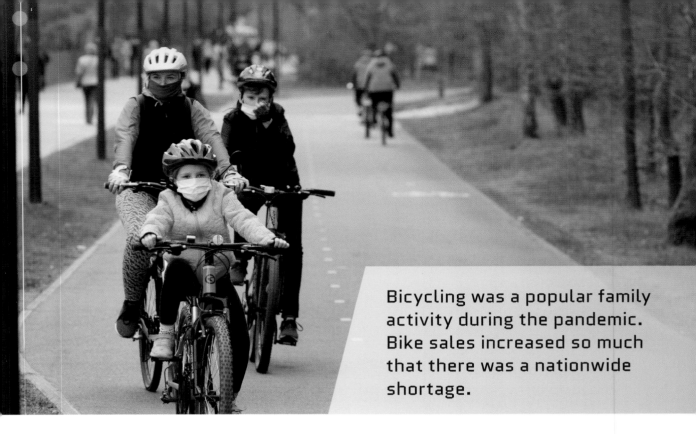

Bicycling was a popular family activity during the pandemic. Bike sales increased so much that there was a nationwide shortage.

They could also do outdoor activities such as biking and walking. However, the **Centers for Disease Control and Prevention (CDC)** encouraged people to practice social distancing. And, the CDC recommended wearing face masks in public.

Stay-at-home orders forced people to adjust to a new way of life. Suddenly, people couldn't go to movie theaters. They couldn't work out at the gym. Kids couldn't go to their friends' houses. To many Americans, life seemed to have changed overnight.

Dining In

Restaurants were among the first businesses to close during the **pandemic.** This was because restaurants often fit many dining tables within a small space. So, it would be easy for COVID-19 to spread among diners.

However, restaurants could still offer take-out and delivery service. Fast food restaurants could also keep their drive-through windows open. These options were safer than dining inside a restaurant. That's because customers could receive their food through little to no contact with others.

FOOD INSECURITY

Even before COVID-19, many American families couldn't afford to buy enough food. This is called food insecurity. The COVID-19 pandemic increased food insecurity for many people. For example, many children relied on school meals for food. When schools were closed, children no longer had access to this food. In response, many school districts set up programs to deliver meals to students' homes.

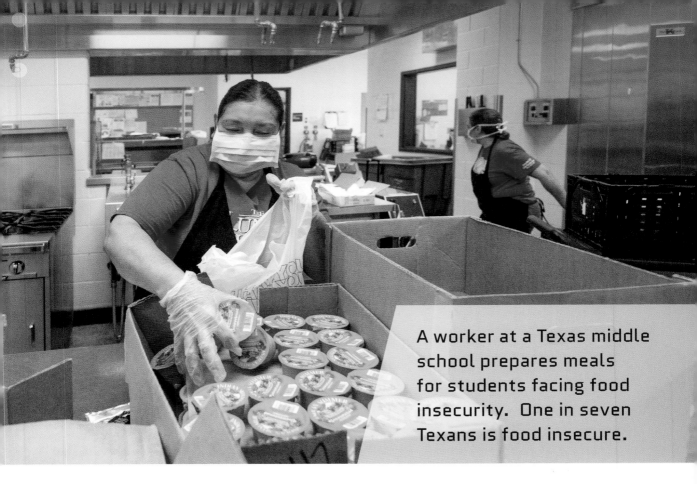

A worker at a Texas middle school prepares meals for students facing food insecurity. One in seven Texans is food insecure.

With restaurants closed, more people cooked and ate meals together than they did before the **pandemic**. This trend had some benefits. For example, home-cooked meals are often healthier than restaurant meals. Also, studies show that eating together can help family members communicate better. Many families found eating together a positive outcome of the pandemic.

Working from Home

The **pandemic** changed how people ate meals. It also changed how people worked. Many workers lost their jobs as businesses closed. But others could work from their homes.

In some ways, working from home was like working in an office. People could still send and receive emails, make phone calls, and do other tasks like normal. One big difference was how meetings were held. People couldn't gather in one room to have a meeting. So, they met online using videoconferencing apps such as Zoom and Microsoft Teams.

Working from home presented both benefits and challenges. Many workers enjoyed not having to commute to their offices. Some were able to keep a **flexible** schedule. However, many workers felt lonely without their co-workers. Workers also reported feeling distracted at home. For many, this meant it took longer to get work done.

Parents working from home also faced challenges. Schools and daycares were closed. So, parents had to work while also watching their children. Many parents could only get work done while their children were napping or sleeping. Because of this, some parents had to work fewer hours. So, they earned less money than normal.

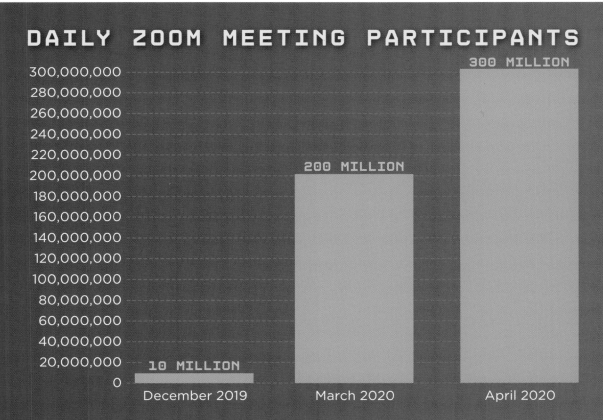

Early in the **pandemic**, more people participated in Zoom meetings than ever before.

Distance Learning

Like workers, students were adjusting to life at home. Most US schools had closed in mid-March 2020. At first, the closures were temporary. But as COVID-19 spread, most schools closed through the end of the school year. With schools closed, students needed another way to complete their studies for the year. Otherwise, they would fall behind in their learning.

Schools offered ways for students to continue learning online. Some teachers emailed students assignments to complete in their own time. Other teachers held virtual lessons using videoconferencing apps.

Distance learning was a solution to schools closing. But it also presented challenges. For example, many lower-income students didn't have access to computers or the internet. So, some school districts worked with computer and internet companies to provide students with this access. And, some cities set up Wi-Fi hot spots to improve internet connections in low-income neighborhoods.

Distance learning also had teachers concerned about their students' well-being. Some children felt scared or anxious about COVID-19. And, some found it difficult to focus during online lessons. Many teachers encouraged students to email them with questions or concerns. In this way, teachers did their best to connect with students from a distance.

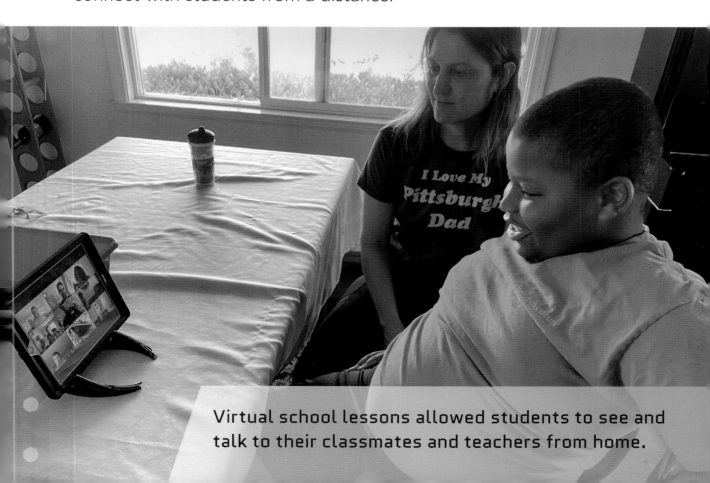

Virtual school lessons allowed students to see and talk to their classmates and teachers from home.

Home for the Holidays

The COVID-19 **pandemic** changed how students experienced school. It also affected many holiday celebrations. During holidays, people would normally get together with loved ones. But during the pandemic, large gatherings were discouraged. So, people celebrated in new ways.

One of the first holidays during the pandemic was St. Patrick's Day on March 17. Cities around the United States canceled their usual St. Patrick's Day parades. The next month brought the religious holidays of Passover, Easter, and Ramadan. Temples, churches, and mosques were closed. So, **congregations** couldn't gather to celebrate and worship together. However, many people still had small celebrations for immediate family members only.

Many states extended their stay-at-home orders into late spring and summer. This affected later holidays. These included Mother's Day, Memorial Day, and the Fourth of July. Instead of having large

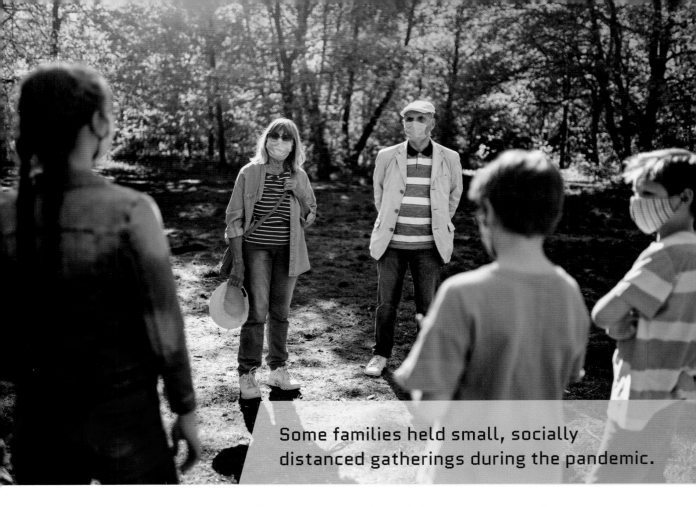

Some families held small, socially distanced gatherings during the pandemic.

picnics or backyard barbecues, people celebrated **remotely**. They talked to family members using video apps such as Facetime, Skype, and Zoom. These tools allowed people to have virtual parties with their loved ones. However, people missed being able to celebrate holidays in person.

Family Events

Holiday gatherings weren't the only large events affected by the COVID-19 **pandemic.** People also couldn't gather as normal for weddings, graduations, and funerals. Many of these events were commemorated **remotely.** Others were **postponed** or modified to follow social distancing guidelines.

Many couples postponed their weddings during the pandemic. Some held ceremonies with just a few family members present.

ASSISTED LIVING FACILITIES

Elderly people were at higher risk of dying from COVID-19. One reason is that elderly people often live in assisted living facilities. It was difficult to maintain social distancing in these places. That's because facility staff had to get close to residents to care for them. To protect the residents, many assisted living facilities didn't allow visitors. If someone wanted to visit a resident, they could stand outside the building and talk through a window.

Eight out of ten Americans killed by COVID-19 were aged 65 years or older.

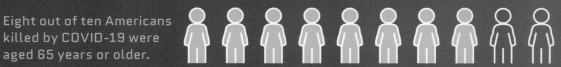

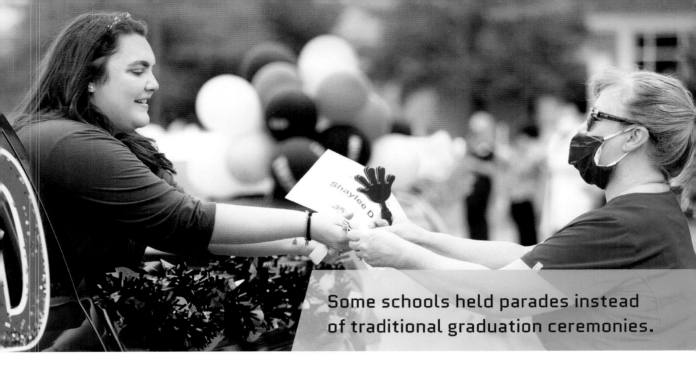

Some schools held parades instead of traditional graduation ceremonies.

Other couples held their weddings virtually. Guests could watch virtual weddings through **livestreams**.

During the **pandemic**, some high schools and colleges canceled their graduation ceremonies. Graduates instead received their **diplomas** in the mail. Other schools allowed graduates to receive their diplomas in small groups. That way, attendees could remain socially distanced.

Some funerals were held in person. But they still needed to follow social distancing guidelines. This often meant limiting the number of people in attendance. Some funerals were livestreamed so people could view the service **remotely**.

Entertainment and Sports

The **pandemic** also affected large entertainment events. Social distancing guidelines and stay-at-home orders meant people couldn't gather in theaters and stadiums. So plays, concerts, and other shows were canceled. Major sporting events were also canceled or **postponed**.

As live events were canceled, more people enjoyed entertainment from home. Production companies released some new movies online. These included *Trolls World Tour* and *Artemis Fowl*. And, musicians recorded performances from their homes. They posted these performances on social media platforms.

Sports fans had more limited options. On March 11, the National Basketball Association suspended its season. The next day, the National Collegiate Athletic Association canceled its athletic championships. These included the popular basketball tournaments known as March Madness.

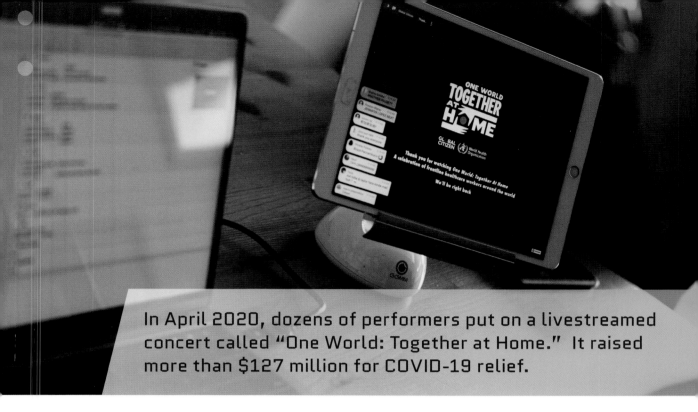

In April 2020, dozens of performers put on a livestreamed concert called "One World: Together at Home." It raised more than $127 million for COVID-19 relief.

International sporting events were also **postponed** or canceled. One was the Summer Olympic Games in Japan. Another was the Wimbledon Tennis Championships in England. With no live sports to air, TV networks showed alternate sports programming. Many stations replayed important games from the past.

Some professional sports returned during the summer. These included baseball, soccer, and basketball. Fans were not allowed to attend games. But they were able to watch live sports on TV again. To many fans, this helped life seem more normal.

Getting Moving

The **pandemic** affected many sports that people liked to watch. It also affected sports that people liked to participate in. Across the country, many sports leagues were canceled. These included baseball, softball, volleyball, and soccer leagues. Golf courses and swimming pools were also closed. And, gyms and fitness studios shut down.

These closures and cancelations forced many people to find new ways to stay active during the pandemic. Some people exercised using online fitness classes. Others bought their own gym equipment so they could work out at home. And, many people turned to outdoor exercise. This included running, hiking,

STEM CONNECTION

The body's immune system is made of cells, tissues, and organs. This system helps fight **infections**. Regular exercise can help strengthen the immune system by increasing the activity of white blood cells. These cells look for and destroy viruses and other germs. For a few hours after exercising, the body is better able to detect and fight germs.

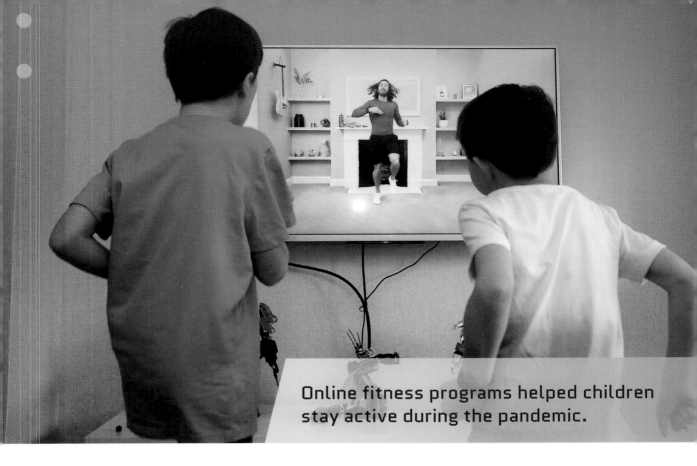

Online fitness programs helped children stay active during the pandemic.

and biking. These were considered safe options because it was easy to practice social distancing while doing them.

Biking became especially popular during the **pandemic**. Bicycle stores across the country reported higher sales than usual. Some people bought new bikes for their whole families. And, one survey found that 21 percent of bike-owning Americans rode more often during the pandemic.

Mental Toll

Over time, Americans adapted to some aspects of life at home. But living under stay-at-home orders was often **stressful**. People felt lonely and **isolated**. Connecting with loved ones through video helped. However, many missed seeing others in person.

People also felt stress due to their financial situation. Many lost their jobs or couldn't work as many hours during the **pandemic**. So, they earned less money.

Those who lost their jobs could apply for their state's unemployment benefits. These benefits provided money for living expenses. But in many cases, these benefits didn't cover all expenses. For example, many Americans struggled to pay their rent or **mortgage**.

On top of the loneliness and stress was a fear of COVID-19 itself. By May 18, more than 1.5 million people in the United States had been **infected**. Nearly 90,000 had died. Many people were afraid they'd catch the virus. People also worried about losing friends and relatives to the disease.

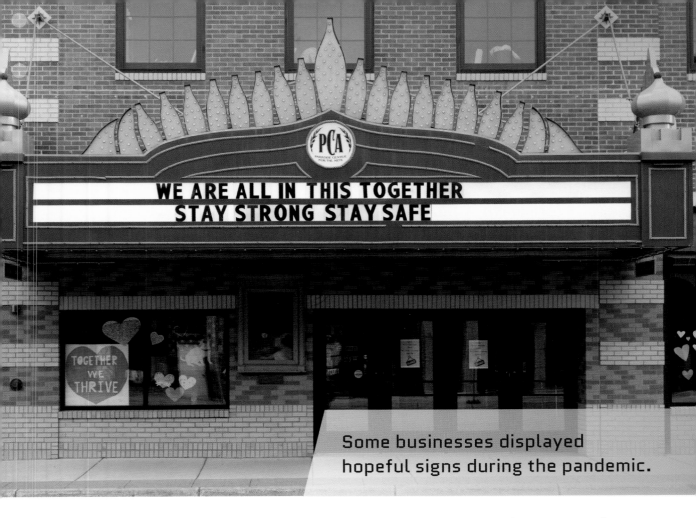

WE ARE ALL IN THIS TOGETHER
STAY STRONG STAY SAFE

PCA
PARADISE CENTER
FOR THE ARTS

TOGETHER WE THRIVE

Some businesses displayed hopeful signs during the pandemic.

Mental health organizations helped people handle the **stress** of living through a **pandemic**. These experts provided tips on how to relax and recover from stress. And, they ran phone lines for people who needed help.

Global Impact

DENMARK

On March 11, Denmark's government asked citizens to limit large gatherings. The country's schools also closed. Three days later, the country closed its borders to foreign travelers. By mid-April, new COVID-19 cases in the country had decreased. So, children returned to schools.

ITALY

Italian citizens were asked to stay at home starting on March 10. On April 14, some **nonessential** businesses, such as bookstores, were allowed to reopen. Customers at these stores had to wear face masks and gloves while shopping. And, workers had to clean their stores twice a day. This was to help kill germs that could spread COVID-19.

TAIWAN

The Taiwanese government never imposed a stay-at-home order. Instead of closing businesses, the government tracked people who had been **infected** with COVID-19. People who encountered infected individuals were asked to stay at home. Citizens were also encouraged to practice social distancing. Most wore face masks in public. And, people had to get their temperatures checked before entering businesses. Anyone with a fever, a **symptom** of COVID-19, was not allowed to enter.

SOUTH AFRICA

On March 26, South Africans were asked to stay at home. Unlike in many countries, outdoor activities were not allowed in South Africa. This included exercising and dog walking. South Africans could only leave their homes to buy food or medicine.

Returning to Normal

In May, COVID-19 cases started declining. So, many states began easing their stay-at-home orders. This meant businesses were allowed to reopen. But **restrictions** weren't lifted completely. In most areas, businesses had to limit the number of people who could be inside. And, social distancing was still encouraged.

Unfortunately, many states that reopened saw a sharp increase in COVID-19 cases. In late June, the governors of some of these states ordered businesses to close again.

As fall approached, so did another school year. So, states had to decide whether to open schools. Some states issued statewide rules that applied to all schools. In other states, the decision was left to each school district.

This led to many different plans across the country. In some areas, students went to school every day. In other areas, students did their schoolwork at home. Many areas used a mix of in-school and at-home learning.

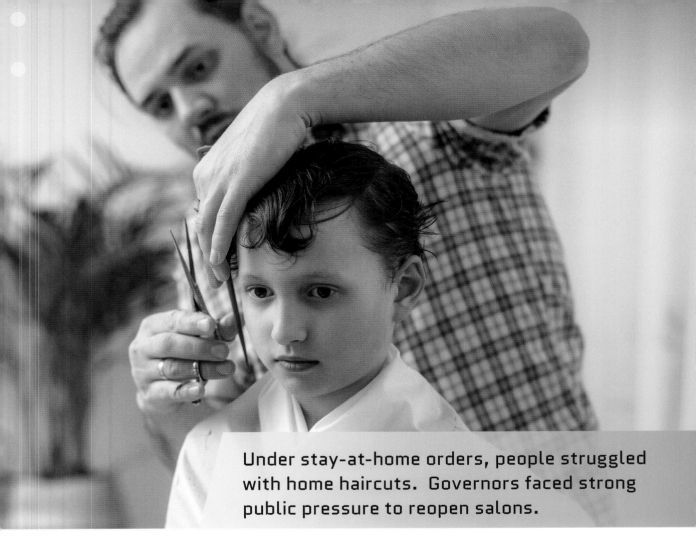

Under stay-at-home orders, people struggled with home haircuts. Governors faced strong public pressure to reopen salons.

The number of COVID-19 cases continued to rise and fall across the country. Citizens and officials were unsure how best to live through the **pandemic**. Only one thing was certain. Returning to normal life would be a long process.

Glossary

Centers for Disease Control and Prevention (CDC)—the main national health organization in the United States. The CDC works to control the spread of disease and maintain and improve public health in the United States and other countries.

congregation—a number of people gathered together, often for worship or religious instruction.

diploma—a certificate showing that a person has graduated from a school.

essential—very important or necessary. Something that is not essential is nonessential.

flexible—easily changed.

infection—an unhealthy condition caused by something harmful, such as a virus. If something has an infection, it is infected.

isolated—separate from others.

livestream—the real-time audio or video transmission of an event over the internet. To transmit such an event is to livestream it.

mortgage (MAWR-gihj)—a legal agreement in which a person borrows money from a financial institution to buy property such as land or a house. He or she pays back the money over a period of years.

pandemic—worldwide spread of a disease that can affect most people.

postpone—to put off until a later time.

remotely—from a distance.

respiratory—having to do with the system of organs involved with breathing.

restriction—a rule that limits or controls something.

stress—a physical, chemical, or emotional factor that causes bodily or mental strain. It may be involved in causing some diseases. Something that causes stress is stressful.

symptom—a noticeable change in the normal working of the body. A symptom indicates or accompanies disease, sickness, or another malfunction.

World Health Organization (WHO)—an agency of the United Nations that works to maintain and improve the health of people around the world.

Online Resources

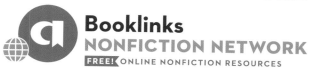

Booklinks
NONFICTION NETWORK
FREE! ONLINE NONFICTION RESOURCES

To learn more about the COVID-19 pandemic, please visit **abdobooklinks.com** or scan this QR code. These links are routinely monitored and updated to provide the most current information available.

Index